Meditation in Yin

CULTIVATING STILLNESS FOR INNER HARMONY AND SERENITY

Tristan St. Reynolds

MEDITATION IN YIN:

Cultivating Stillness For Inner Harmony and Serenity

By

TRISTAN ST. REYNOLDS

About the Author:

Tristan St. Reynolds is a versatile Australian talent, celebrated as a Model, Author, and Ambassador. Yet, it's his connection to Yin Yoga and meditation that truly sets him apart. With an extensive background in Yoga, boasting over 2000 hours of training and mentorship from renowned institutions like Essence of Living, Fireshaper, Yoga Alliance Australia and various others. Tristan has evolved into a distinguished Fitness Professional.

In addition to his physical passions, Tristan is a qualified Meditation Facilitator and Transformation Academy Life and Relationship Coach, demonstrating his commitment to guiding individuals towards their highest potential.

Tristan's creative journey extends beyond the mat and meditation cushion. He introduced the world to his first Oracle deck, "Cryptid Whispers," in 2023, a special gift rooted in his journey and to assist others. This innovative creation, along with his compelling children's book, "Finn Finds Home: A Mertail," available on Amazon, exemplifies Tristan's dedication to nurturing the inner selves of all ages.

His influence doesn't stop there. Tristan has made memorable appearances in advertising campaigns and worked at many different facilities.

In 2023, Tristan graced the cover of Marika Magazine, further showcasing his reach and commitment as a guiding force in the realms of mind-body-spirit and wellness. His endeavors in the realm of spirituality, yoga, and holistic well-being have been recognized and celebrated in various ways, affirming his desire to share in wisdom and transformation.

Linktree:

https://linktr.ee/tristanstreynolds

Table of Contents

Introduction

Are you ready to open the door to deep relaxation, increased flexibility, and a deeper connection to your inner self? Look no further than the transforming power of Yin Yoga.

Imagine a yoga practice where gentle meditative poses help release stress, calm your body, and calm your mind. Yin Yoga gives you just that: a peaceful haven in a rapidly changing world. It's a sanctuary where time seems to slow down, allowing you to sink into poses that target the deepest layers of your body. The benefits of this ancient and peaceful art go beyond the physical. As you perform each pose, you embark on a spiritual adventure, unlocking your chakras and tapping into your inner energy centers. It's not just a workout; it is a journey of self-awareness, tuning in to your mind, body, and soul. Yin Yoga is the gateway to a life-changing journey of self-discovery and holistic wellness.

So why wait to experience the deep transfiguration that Yin Yoga can bring to your life? In this book, you will discover the magic of calmness, the power of breathing, and the serenity within you. Embrace the stillness revolution of Yin Yoga today and embark on a journey that will help you revive, balance, and be spiritually awakened. Don't miss the opportunity to redefine your happiness and life. Yin Yoga is the path that leads you to a more active, focused, and harmonious being.

As you read, recall that Yin Yoga is not about perfection; it's a question of progress. Be patient, practice with an open mind, and let each page accompany you on your course to a healthier and more balanced life. So let's begin on this journey together, to the heart of Yin Yoga, where you will discover the ageless wisdom and inner peace that await you.

Chapter 1

Introducing Yin Yoga

Yin yoga is a practice that pushes the boundaries of customary yoga styles. While many yoga styles emphasize dynamism and muscle engagement, Yin Yoga proffer a completely different approach to physical and mental fitness. In this chapter, we will delve deeper into the foundations of Yin Yoga, exploring its unique attributes and ability to change your life.

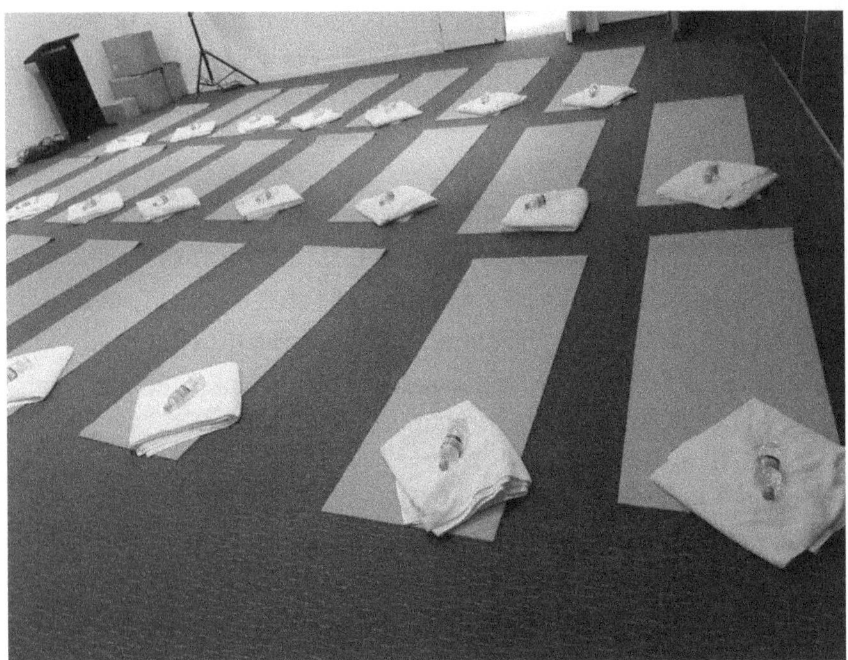

The Nature of Yin Yoga

At its core, Yin Yoga is a slow meditation practice that centers on holding poses for long periods of time. Unlike more energetic styles like Vinyasa or Ashtanga, where you move from one pose to the next in a sequential sequence, Yin Yoga urges you to find calmness in each pose. This quietness allows you to access the body's deeper tissues, including tendons, ligaments, and fascia.

This practice takes its name from the notion of Yin and Yang, a constituent of Chinese philosophy. In this creed, Yin depicts the passive, receptive, and cooling qualities, while Yang represents the active, dynamic, and warm aspects.

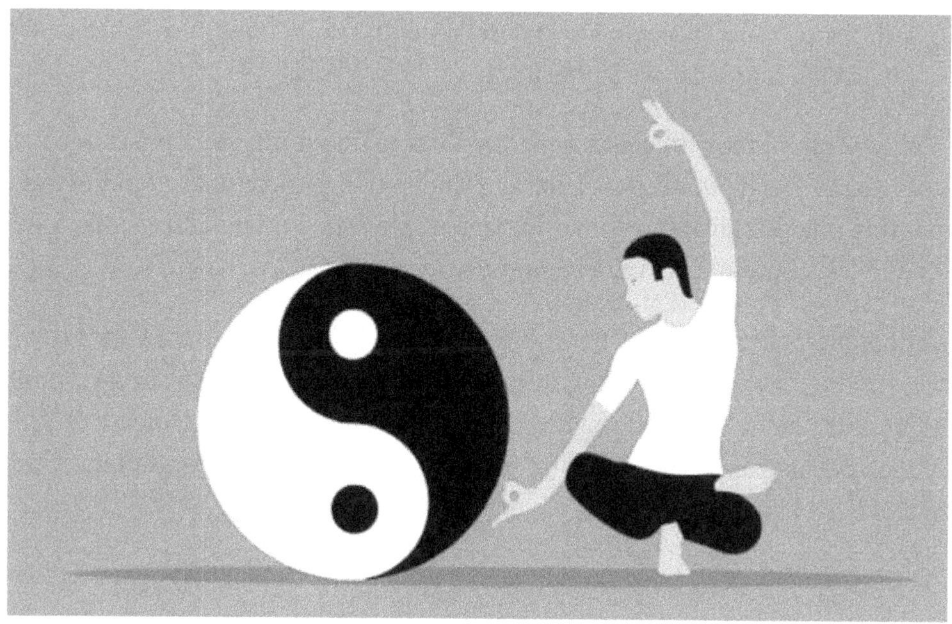

Yin Yoga helps to balance these two opposing forces. Mindfulness is at the heart of Yin Yoga. By holding the pose for long periods of time, you have the chance to observe your sensations, thoughts, and emotions. Self-awareness and being in the present moment are at the heart of the practice. It's not just about stretching your body; it's about stretching your mind and soul.

History of Yin Yoga

Yin Yoga is not just a modern trend; Its roots lie deep in ancient traditions. Yin Yoga has its roots in Taoism, an ancient Chinese philosophy and religion. Taoism believes in the balance of Yin and Yang forces, similar to the principles behind Yin Yoga. In the Taoist tradition, Yin depicts the passive, immobile, and feminine qualities, while Yang represents the active, energetic, and masculine aspects.

The concept of Yin and Yang is essential to understanding the ideology behind Yin Yoga. Balance between these opposing forces is imperative for physical, mental, and spiritual harmony. Taoism instructs that by applying Yin qualities, we can find calmness, acceptance, and inner peace.

While Yin Yoga's philosophical origins date back to ancient times, its modern development can be traced back to Paulie Zin, a martial artist and yoga teacher. In the 1970s, he combined his widespread knowledge of martial arts, including Taoist yoga and

Tai Chi, with the practice of yoga. He created a unique combination of these disciplines, ultimately evolving into what we know today as "Yin Yoga."

Paulie Zink's innovative approach involves maintaining yoga poses for long periods of time to reach the deepest layers of the body and clear energy pathways. He found that this practice had a profound impact on physical and mental health. Yin Yoga was born and has continuously developed over the years.

Although Paulie Zink laid the foundation for Yin Yoga, Bernie Clark is oftentimes credited with popularizing it. Clark's expansive knowledge and commitment to spreading this practice steered the publication of "The Complete Guide to Yin Yoga," a book which became a seminal work on Yin Yoga, aiding people around the world embrace this life-changing practice.

Today, Yin Yoga is an acknowledged and respected form of yoga, practiced by countless people seeking a slower, more meditative activity. It has become popular not only for its physical benefits but also for its ability to calm the mind and bring about deep relaxation.

As you progress through this book, you will develop a better understanding of how these ancient concepts and present-day interpretations have come together to produce a practice that is capable of bringing balance, harmony, and wellness into your life.

Unleashing your inner peace: The powerful world of Yin Yoga and meditation

In a world filled with chaos and constant movement, the connection between Yin Yoga and meditation provides a powerful light of serenity and self-discovery. These two ancient practices weave together to bring about a deep journey of inner peace and overall wellness.

Yin Yoga, with its gentle and thoughtful postures, invites you to pause and listen to the whispers of your body. It is a practice of patience, as you hold a pose for long periods of time, allowing your muscles to relax and your muscles to release. But Yin Yoga is more than simply physical exertion; it is the gateway to meditation in motion. The calmness it develops in your body prepares you to delve into the stillness of your mind.

For its part, meditation is the art of finding inner peace. It is a practice that encourages you to dig into your inner world, cultivating mindfulness and awareness.

When you sit or lie in a meditative state, you begin a journey of self-discovery, gradually peeling away the layers of mental chatter to reveal the quiet core of who you are.

Yin Yoga and meditation together create a harmonious step. Here's how they supplement each other:

i. **Physical and mental liberation:** Yin Yoga prepares your body for meditation by releasing physical tension. As your muscles relax, your mind will follow suit, making it easier for you to meditate with a calm, open awareness.

ii. **Presence and awareness:** Both activities emphasize being available in the present moment. In Yin Yoga, you are fully engaged in the sensations of each pose, while meditation enhances your presence by focusing on your breathing or a specific focus point.

iii. **Energy balance:** Yin Yoga helps balance the body's energy by targeting the meridians and chakras. This paves the way for meditation to balance the mind's energies, promoting mental clarity and inner harmony.

iv. **Strengthening your spiritual journey:** The partnership of Yin Yoga and meditation can open up spiritual dimensions. As your body and mind return to calm, you will be able to experience moments of transcendence and clarity, connecting with your higher self.

Whether you are a seasoned practitioner or a beginner, the combination of Yin Yoga and meditation can bring profound change to your health. Together, they offer the path to a more focused, peaceful, and spiritually awakened life. This symbiotic connection provides the medium needed to quiet the mind, open the heart, and get into an endless source of inner peace.

The Link Between Yin Yoga, Spirituality and Meditation

Yin Yoga is a slow, passive style of yoga that includes holding poses for long periods of time, typically lasting 1–5 minutes. It promotes spirituality and meditation through a peculiar approach to asana practice and its relation to the chakra system. Read on to see how Yin Yoga can enrich your spiritual and meditative journey, focusing on the chakras it unlocks.

Yin Yoga and Chakras:

Yin Yoga is deeply connected to the philosophy of chakras, which are the energy centers of the body. Practicing Yin Yoga can help unlock and balance these chakras, which in turn can enrich your spiritual and meditative experiences.

Root Chakra (Muladhara):

The first chakra, located at the base of the spine, controls our feelings of safety and security. Yin poses such as "Butterfly" or "Sphinx" can help level and stabilize this chakra. When the root chakra is balanced, it can lay a solid foundation for your spiritual growth and meditation practice.

Sacral Chakra (Svadhisthana):

The sacral chakra, located in the lower abdomen, is related to emotions and creativity. Yin poses such as "Dragon" and "Butterfly" can stimulate this chakra, allowing for a deeper connection to your emotions and inner creative energy.

Solar Plexus Chakra (Manipura):

This chakra, located in the upper abdomen, is associated with personal power and confidence. Poses like "Twisted Root" and "Banana" in Yin Yoga can help activate and balance the solar plexus chakra, strengthening self-esteem and mental strength.

Heart Chakra (Anahata):

The heart chakra, located in the middle of the chest, is associated with love and compassion. Yin poses such as "Melting Heart" and "Saddle" open and heal this chakra, promoting feelings of love, empathy, and deeper connection with others and oneself.

Throat Chakra (Vishuddha):

The throat chakra is responsible for communication and self-expression. Yin Yoga poses like "Cat Pulling Tail" and "Swan" can activate and balance this chakra, helping you express your true self and enhance your meditation experience.

Third Eye Chakra (Ajna):

The third eye chakra, located between the eyebrows, is associated with intuition and insight. Poses like "Children's Pose" and "Dragonfly" can stimulate this chakra, helping to enhance your meditation and inner awareness.

Crown Chakra (Sahasrara):

The crown chakra, at the top of the head, interconnects with enlightenment and spiritual unity. Yin Yoga poses that promote feelings of surrender and liberation, such as "Shavasana" and "Corpse Pose," can help you access higher states of consciousness and connect with your spiritual self.

The slow, passive nature of Yin Yoga allows you to dig into these chakras and their related qualities with greater depth and awareness. When incorporated with focused breathing and mindfulness, it can significantly enrich your spiritual journey and meditation practice, promoting a sense of balance, inner peace, and connection to your higher self. It is significant to note that the effects of Yin yoga on the chakras can differ from person to person, and consistency in practice is essential to benefiting from these assets.

Chapter 2

Why do people practice Yin Yoga

People are drawn to Yin Yoga for a myriad of reasons, and in this chapter, I will walk you through the different motivations that lead individuals to start practicing. Yin Yoga has something to offer anyone, whether you are looking for physical relaxation, mental stillness, or a deep mind-body affinity.

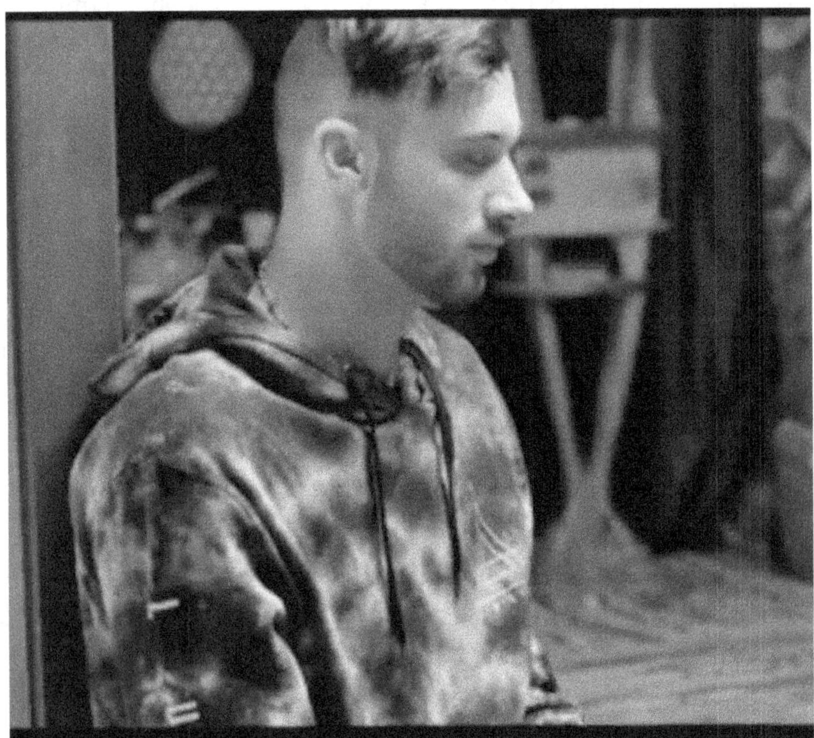

Below are some of the reasons to practice Yin Yoga:

i. **Improving joint health:** Yin Yoga may be especially beneficial for your joint health. You can minimize stiffness and prevent age-related challenges like arthritis by gently stretching and releasing the connective tissue around your joints. For those with joint issues, Yin Yoga can help reduce pain and improve mobility.

ii. **Improving posture:** Good posture is critical for maintaining a healthy spine and overall health. Yin Yoga emboldens alignment and body awareness, aiding you to maintain better posture in everyday life. This can be particularly useful for people who spend many hours sitting at a desk.

iii. **Improving circulation:** Gentle stretches and sustaining Yin Yoga positions can improve blood circulation. It promotes blood flow to distinct areas of the body, which can lead to improved tissue oxygenation and better overall health.

iv. **Reducing stress and tension:** As Yin Yoga promotes relaxation and calm, it can considerably reduce stress and tension in the body. Stress is often evident physically as muscle and joint tension. Yin Yoga helps release these physical embodiment of tension, leading to better relaxation and wellness.

v. **Improving organ functions:** The stretches and pressure applied to given areas in Yin Yoga poses can energize and massage the internal organs. This gentle massage effect can improve organ function and enhance overall health.

vi. **Improving energy flow:** In Chinese medicine, the notion of energy flow or "chi" is essential. Yin Yoga aids in clearing blockages in the body's energy pathways, allowing energy to flow more easily. This can lead to better vitality and a greater feeling of wellness.

vii. **Preventing and controlling chronic pain:** Yin Yoga can be a helpful tool for people with chronic pain like back pain, hip pain, or joint pain. Gently stretching and releasing tension in distinct areas can offer pain relief and help address chronic discomfort.

viii. **Improving athletic performance:** Athletes usually ascertain that Yin Yoga can complement their regular exercise programs, as it enhances flexibility, reduces the risk of injury, and accelerates recovery. By integrating Yin Yoga into their program, athletes can improve their overall performance.

ix. **Recovery after exertion:** If you are recovering from exertion or injury, Yin Yoga can be a delicate yet effective recovery method. Passive stretching and a slower pace give your body the care it requires to heal and reclaim strength without overexertion.

x. **Connecting the mind and body:** For those looking for a stronger mind-body connection, Yin Yoga provides a route to self-discovery. By practicing and doing calming poses, you will learn to listen to your body and mind with more rapt. This amplified awareness can lead to a deeper sense of self and inner harmony.

xi. **Deeper relaxation:** Yin Yoga is a deep relaxation practice that gives respite from the bustling pace of modern life. People who struggle to relax and let go of stress often turn to Yin Yoga for its competence to induce a state of deep relaxation.

xii. Many people suffer from sleep disorders and insomnia. The relaxation and stress reduction benefits of Yin Yoga can lead to better quality sleep. By calming the nervous system and reducing mental stress, Yin Yoga can aid you enjoy a better night's sleep.

xiii. Yin Yoga's underscoring on mindfulness can have a significant impact on mental health. The practice can help manage anxiety, depression, and other emotional issues. It teaches you to accept the present moment and acquire resilience in the face of adversity.

xiv. In the fast-paced society of today, Yin Yoga offers the room to let go of expectations and aims. It's not about striving for a specific pose or perfect alignment. It's about ceding to the present moment and accepting yourself as you are.

Chapter 3

Yin Yoga and Other Styles

Yin Yoga does not exist in a vacuum; it may supplement and enrich your experience with other types of yoga. In this chapter, we'll look at ways you can integrate Yin Yoga into your present yoga practice or utilize it as a stand-alone road to well-being.

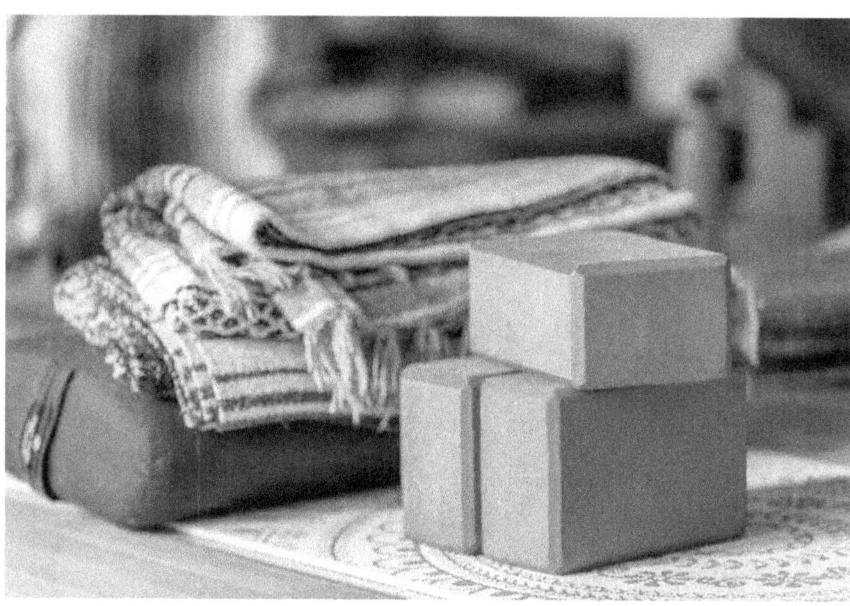

The Yin Yoga Sequence

A typical Yin Yoga session includes a series of poses that target distinct areas of the body. These positions can vary, but in general they include backward bends, forward bends, twists, and hip openers. Each pose lasts a certain amount of time, allowing you to examine and experience the unique feeling of each pose.

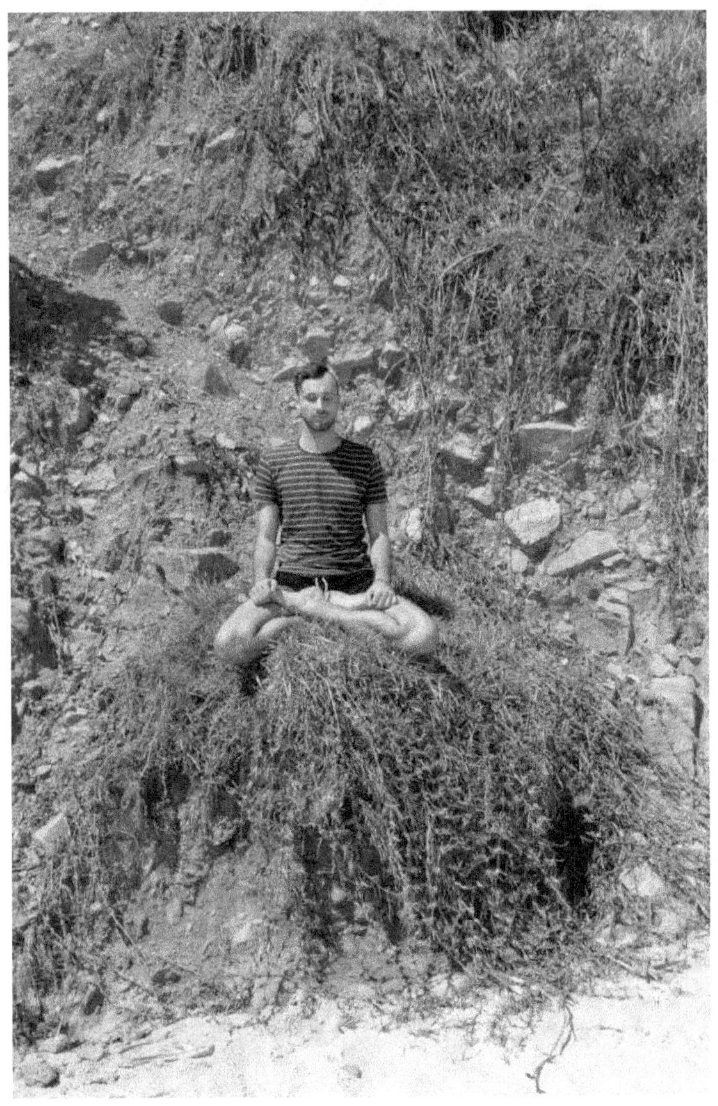

Common poses for your sequencing

Healing Benefit: Eases tension in the hips and groin, aids in emotional release, and supports hip flexibility.

Passive Bridge (with block or bolster):

Yin Benefit: Opens the chest, stretches the spine, and provides a gentle backbend.

Healing Benefit: Relieves lower back discomfort, supports respiratory function, and encourages a sense of expansion.

Passive Shoulder Stand:

Yin Benefit: Promotes a gentle inversion, offering a soothing effect on the nervous system.

Healing Benefit: Improves blood circulation, reduces stress, and supports thyroid function.

Savasana:

Yin Benefit: Offers complete relaxation, allowing the body to absorb the benefits of the practice.

Healing Benefit: Facilitates deep rest, reduces stress, and supports mental and emotional rejuvenation.

These poses are often incorporated into Yin yoga practices, which focus on longer holds and passive stretches to target deeper connective tissues. This approach promotes relaxation and healing by gently stressing the tissues and encouraging the release of tension.

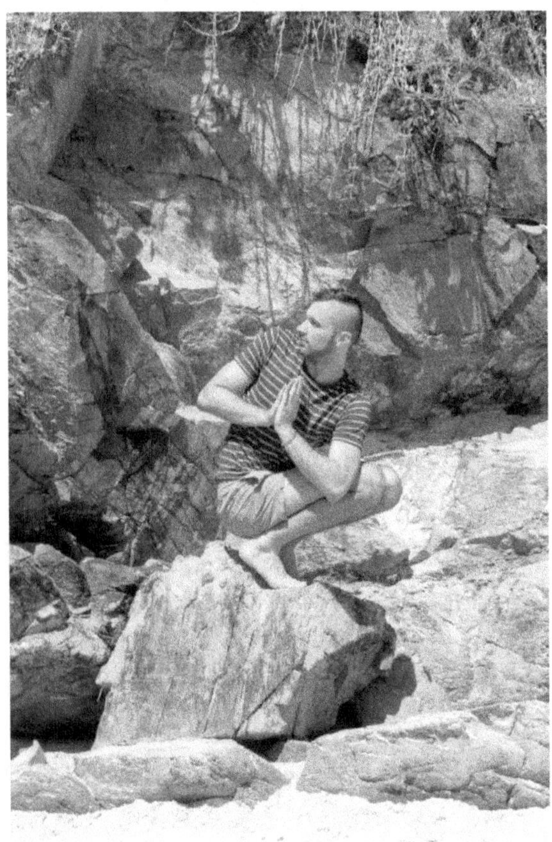

Finding balance in your practice

Many people are drawn to yoga because of its diverse nature. Yoga offers a variety of styles, from vigorous and dynamic to slow and meditative. While Yin Yoga and more Yang-oriented styles each have their own benefits, it's important to find the right balance for your individual needs. Integrating Yin Yoga into your practice can give a much-needed counterbalance to more energetic styles. If you are a devoted Ashtanga or Vinyasa practitioner, the calmness of Yin Yoga can give you the opportunity to slow down, stretch deeply, and unfold a profound connection between mind and body. Yin

Yoga as a practice of self-mastery

Yin Yoga can also be a complete and independent practice. If you are new to yoga or simply find the lightness and stillness of Yin Yoga appealing, you can make it your main yoga practice. You don't need any previous experience with other styles of yoga to fully grasp Yin Yoga.

Combining Yin and Yang

Some yoga devotee choose to alternate Yin and Yang exercises. For example, you could take a dynamic Vinyasa class one day and follow it up with a calming Yin session the next. This balance permit you to dig into the best of both worlds, promoting flexibility, strength and mental peace.

Your body's needs changes daily. Some days, you may crave the restorative energy of a Yang practice, while other days, the calm and relaxation of Yin Yoga may be just what you need. By heeding to your body, you can adjudge which style best suits your current state.

Incorporating Yin postures

During a Yang yoga class, you can seamlessly incorporate Yin Yoga poses to improve your experience. After a dynamic sequence, incorporating several Yin poses can aid release tension and promote a feeling of relaxation. Poses like Sphinx, Butterfly, or Sleeping Swan can be incorporated into your regular yoga practice.

Yin Pose	Rebound Pose
Puppy Pose	Child's Pose
Baddha Konasana	Reclined Butterfly
Half Butterfly	Reclined Tree
Caterpillar	Supported Fish
Deer	Reclined Tree
Dragon	Reclined Swan
Sleep Swan	Child's Pose
Sphinx	Crocodile

The power of Yin Yoga poses

In this section, we'll take a deeper look at some of the key Yin Yoga poses and explore how each pose can work specific areas of your body and mind. These poses are the foundation of your Yin Yoga practice, and understanding their benefits is essential to a well-rounded practice.

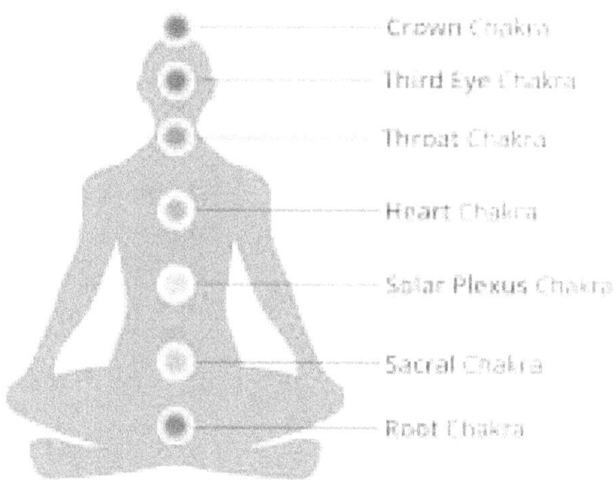

Butterfly pose (Baddha Konasana)

Benefits: The butterfly pose is a great pose to open the hips and groin. It stretches the inner thighs and can relieve sciatica. This pose is deeply soothing and helps reduce stress and anxiety.

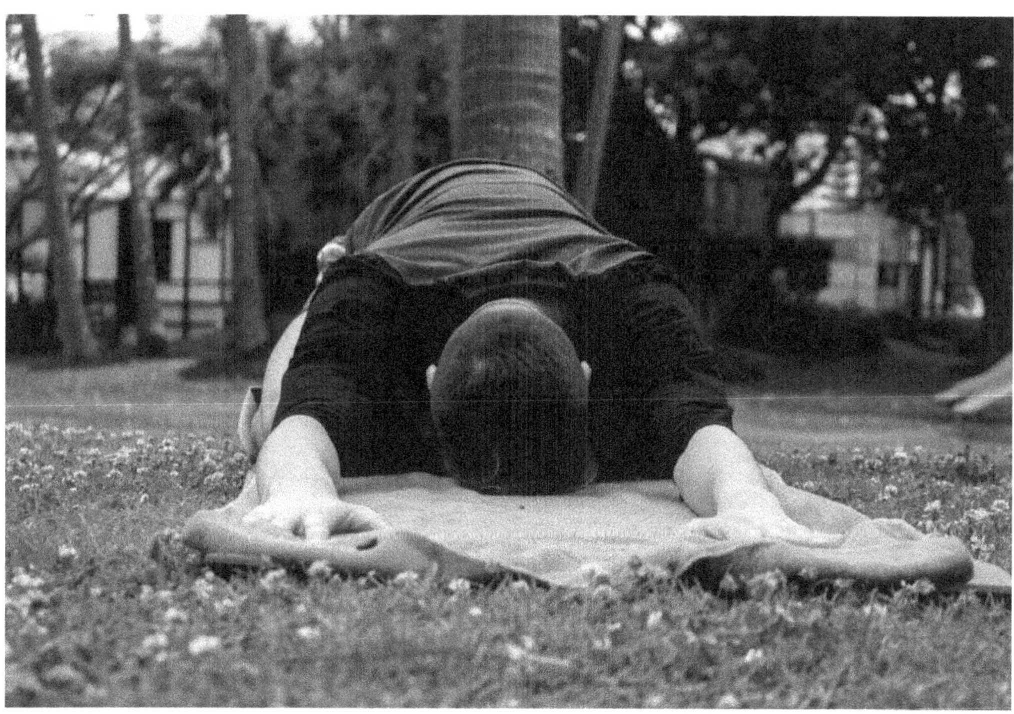

Child's Pose (Balasana)

Benefits: A child's pose is a resting and grounding position. It gently stretches your lower back, hips, and thighs. This is an ideal position for relaxation and can reduce stress and fatigue.

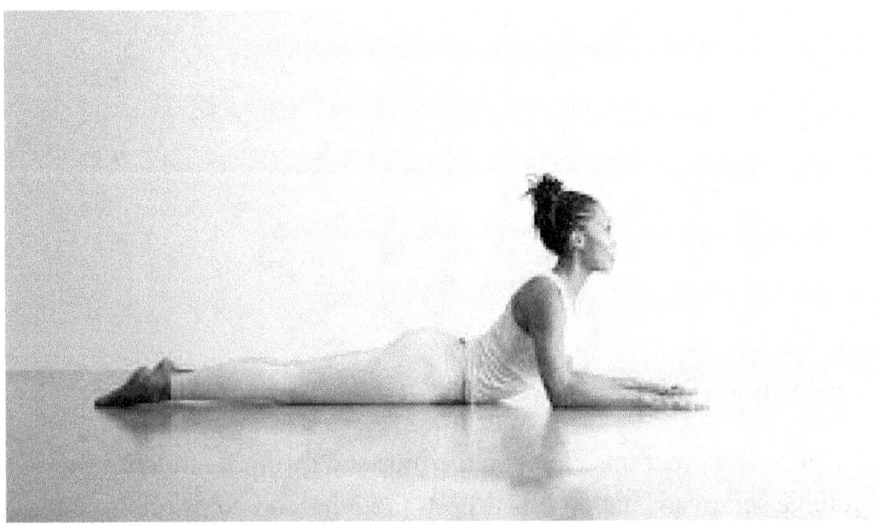

Sphinx pose:

Benefits: Sphinx pose is great for opening the chest and stretching the abdominal muscles. This can help relieve back pain and promote a feeling of emotional release. This is great for people who spend long hours sitting at a desk.

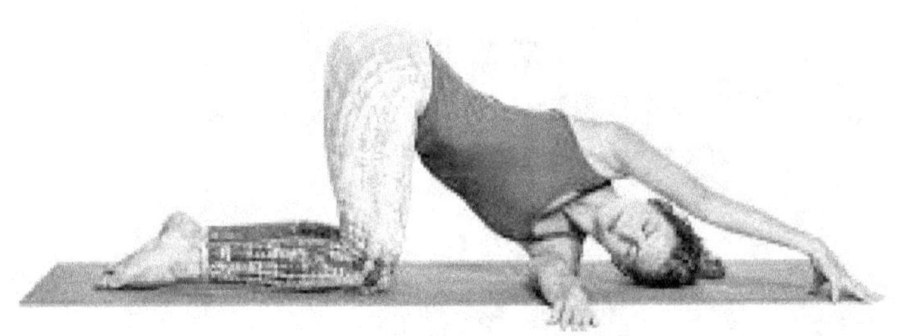

Needle Threading Pose (Parsva Balasana)

Benefits: This pose targets the shoulders and upper back. It can help enhance spinal flexibility and reduce tension in the neck and shoulders. This is particularly beneficial for people with sedentary jobs.

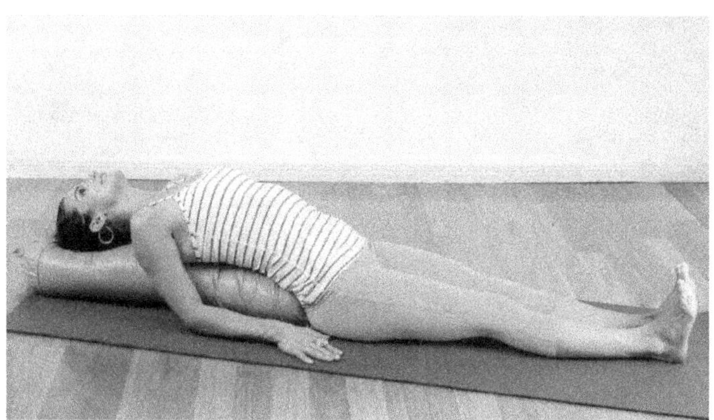

Supported fish pose (Matsyasana variation)

Benefits: The supported fish pose is a heart-opening pose that stretches and relaxes the chest and shoulders. This is a great position for people who spend a lot of time sitting in front of a screen or desk.

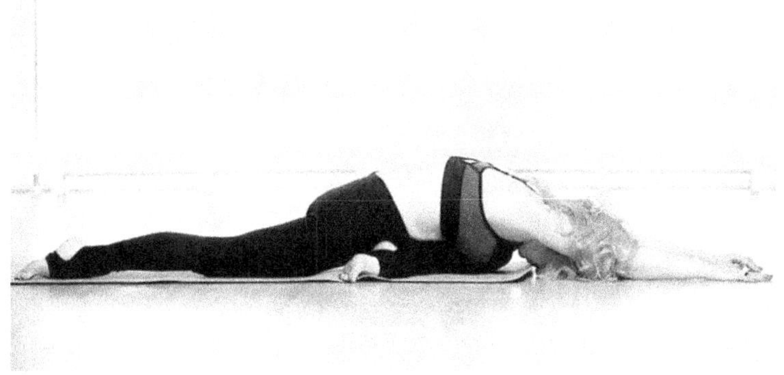

Sleeping Swan Pose (Pigeon Pose)

Benefits: The Sleeping Swan Pose is a deep hip-opening exercise. It can help release emotions and tension built up in the hips, making it a favorite sport for those looking for emotional and physical release.

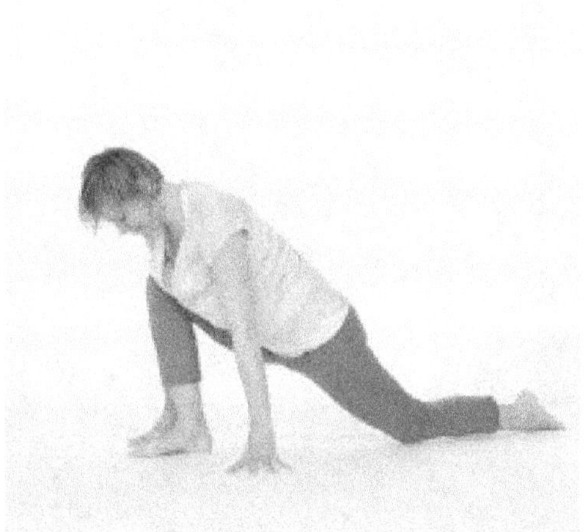

Dragon pose

Benefits: Dragon pose deeply stretches the hip flexors and groin. This is great for athletes and people with tight hips. Regular exercise can improve hip flexibility and prevent lower back pain.

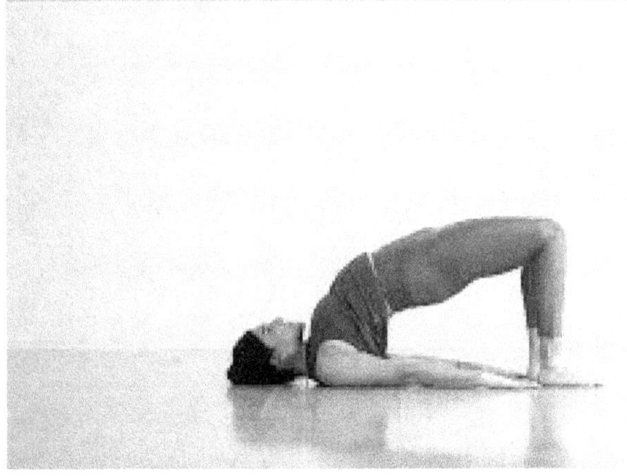

Supported Bridge Pose

Benefits: The supported bridge pose provides a gentle stretch to the spine and front of the body. It can soothe back pain and reduce stress. This pose is suitable for people who want to experience a mild inversion without much effort.

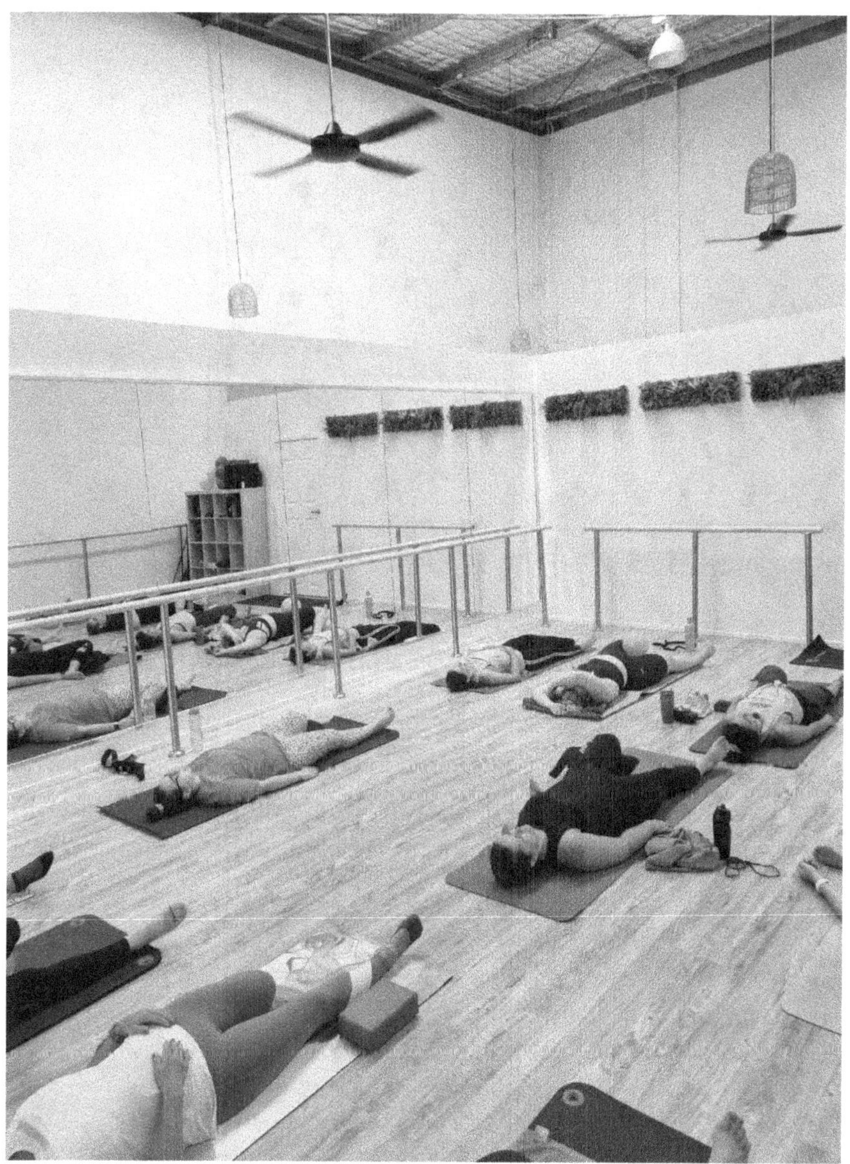

Savasana (corpse pose)

Benefits: Savasana is the maximum relaxation pose and an essential part of any yoga practice. It helps the body and mind assimilate the benefits of your practice and is great for stress reduction and deep relaxation.

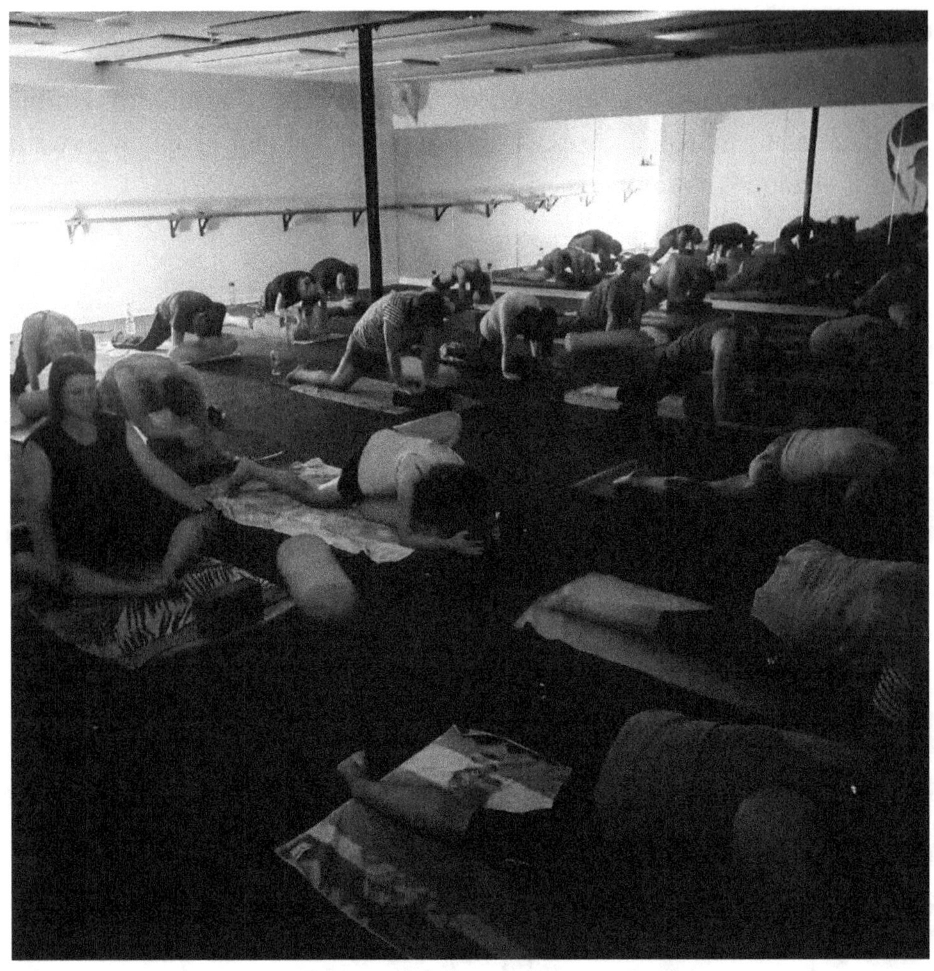

Remember, Yin Yoga poses are not about achieving extreme flexibility or pushing your limits. It's about finding your edge, staying calm, and allowing your body to gradually open up over time. Each pose has its own benefits, and together they breed a practice that promotes deep release, flexibility, and emotional wellness.

Conclusion

Throughout this book, we've examined the world of Yin Yoga, from its historical origins to its esoteric physical, emotional, and psychological benefits. Yin Yoga is more than just a bodily practice; it is a path towards self-discovery, balance, and happiness.

Yin Yoga's unique approach to stillness, mindfulness, and gentle stretching makes it the ideal practice for those looking to reduce stress, improve flexibility, balance emotions, and improve mental clarity. Whether you are a seasoned practitioner or new to the world of yoga, Yin Yoga offers something for everyone.

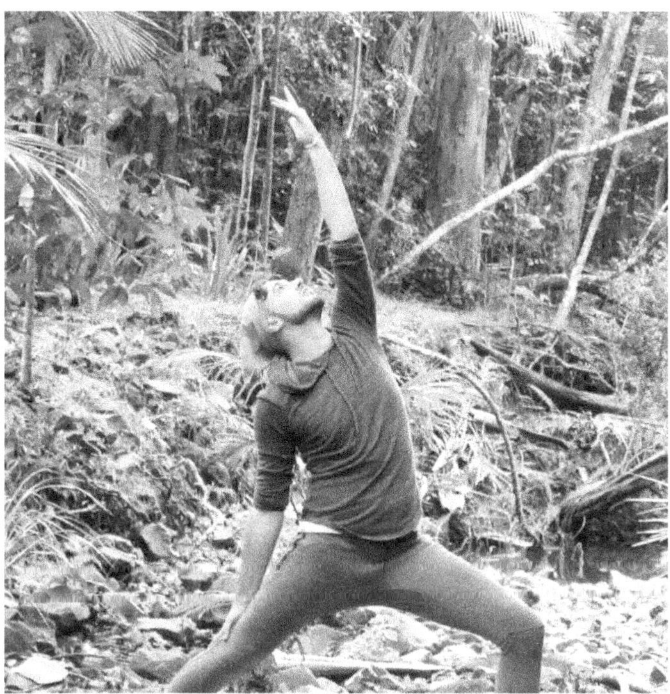

By applying the principles of Yin Yoga and integrating its postures and practices into your life, you can experience an immense transfiguration that goes far beyond the yoga mat. Yin Yoga is an invitation to delve into the depths of your body and mind, providing a holistic approach to well-being.

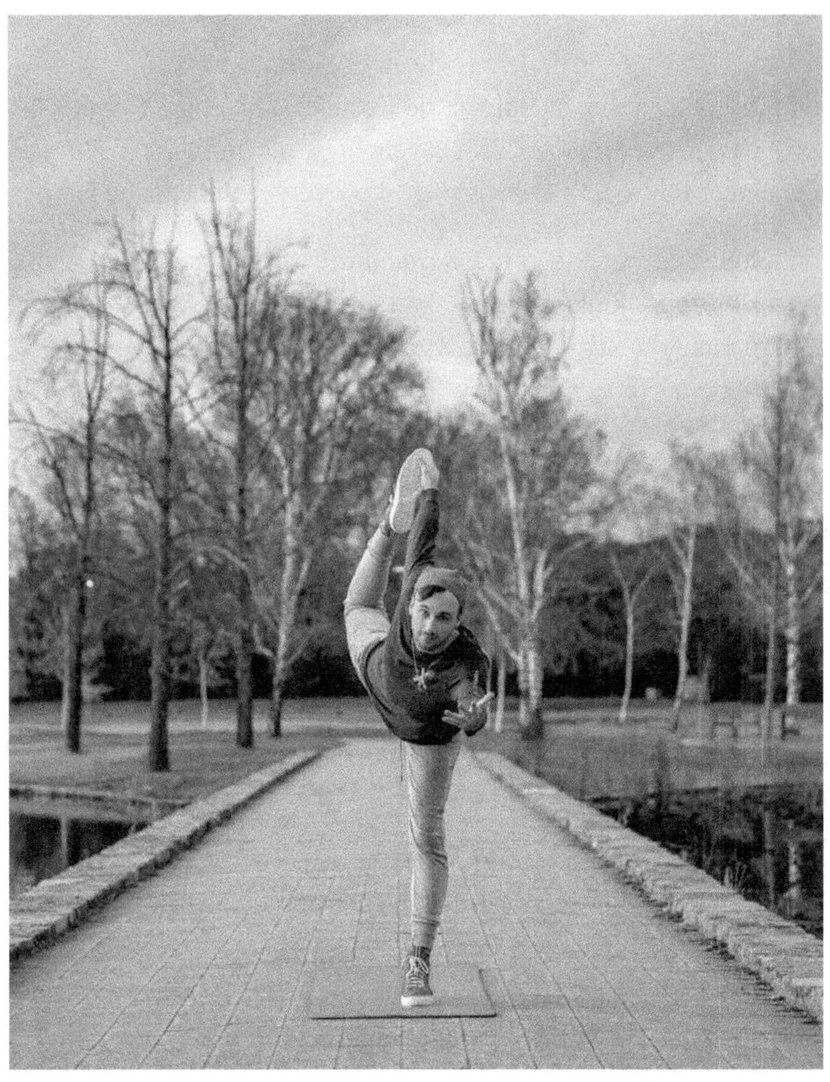

As you continue your expedition with Yin Yoga, remember that this exercise is not about perfection; it's a quest for progress. Have your moment, be patient with yourself, and allow each pose and breath to guide you toward better health.

Closing Message:

"In my extensive Yoga training and years of teaching Yoga, I've come to understand the profound nature of stillness and movement in healing both the mind and body. Yin Yoga, in particular, has gifted me with a deep sense of grounding, unwavering focus, physical relief, and mental clarity.

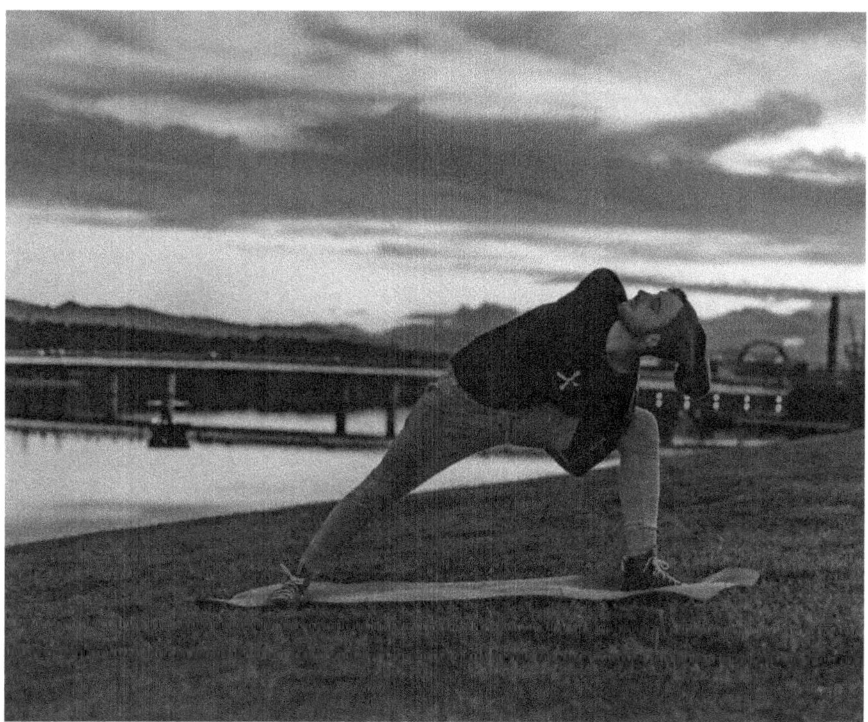

I believe, much like in yogic, tantric, and vedic philosophy, that there is a balance of light and dark within each of us. The idea of Yin and Yang. Balance is a gift from God. Sharing Yoga is more than a profession; it transcends being able to exercise. It's a nurturing of one's spirit, a special journey. I am grateful for the privilege of witnessing people's deepest struggles and seeing them towards a transformative exchange, where a little piece of light can replace the shadows.

I hold a deep reverence for the energy that flows within us—it is both special and sacred. Embrace the passage of time, allowing yourself to feel every moment in your body. Listen intently to the whispers of your heart, and let them be your guiding light, synchronized with the rhythm of your breath and the luminance of your soul."

-- Tristan St. Reynolds

References

1. Campbell, Roger J. "Yin Yoga: Stretch the Mind, Free the Body." Penguin, 2012.

2. Clark, Bernie. "The Complete Guide to Yin Yoga." White Cloud Press, 2012.

3. Farhi, Donna. "The Breathing Book: Good Health and Vitality Through Essential Breath Work." Holt Paperbacks, 1996.

4. Gannon, Sharon, and David Life. "Jivamukti Yoga: Practices for Liberating Body and Soul." Ballantine Books, 2002.

5. Grilley, Paul. "Yin Yoga: Principles and Practice." Pranamaya, 2002.

6. Grilley, Paul. "Yin Yoga: Outline of a Quiet Practice." White Cloud Press, 2002.

7. Jivamukti Yoga School. "The Art of Yoga." Stewart, Tabori & Chang, 2002.

8. Kaminoff, Leslie, and Amy Matthews. "Yoga Anatomy." Human Kinetics, 2007.

9. Lasater, Judith Hanson. "Relax and Renew: Restful Yoga for Stressful Times." Rodmell Press, 2011.

10. McCall, Timothy. "Yoga as Medicine: The Yogic Prescription for Health and Healing." Bantam, 2007.

11. Powers, Sarah. "Insight Yoga." Shambhala Publications, 2008.

12. Satchidananda, Swami. "The Yoga Sutras of Patanjali." Integral Yoga Publications, 2012.